contents

1. Introduction to First Aid

Learning how to react to medical crises and provide first treatment to an injured or unwell individual requires a thorough understanding of first aid. First aid is the emergency treatment provided to a person after they have been hurt or become unexpectedly unwell before professional medical assistance arrives.

The quick treatment provided to someone who has been hurt or becomes sick without warning is known as first aid. First aid aims to maintain life, stop an accident or sickness from growing worse, and hasten recovery. In an emergency, first aid is often the first line of defense and may have a big impact on how an accident or disease turns out.

Everyone should be able to execute basic first aid procedures since accidents and emergencies may occur at any time and anyplace. Cuts and scratches, burns, fractured bones, choking, heart attacks, and allergic responses are a few instances when first aid may be required.

First aid is meant to keep people alive, stop their condition from becoming worse, and encourage recovery. initial aid administered correctly may have a big impact on how things turn out in the crucial initial few minutes after an illness or accident.

Regardless of career or experience, it is important for everyone to learn the fundamentals of first aid. It may help save lives by enabling people to react to medical crises swiftly and efficiently.

The basic steps and methods of first aid, such as CPR, using an AED, and providing first aid for particular injuries and medical crises, will be covered in this first aid manual. We will also go over how to improve health and avoid accidents, as well as how to be prepared for disasters.

By the time you finish reading this manual, you will have a fundamental grasp of first aid concepts and techniques, and you will be better prepared to react to medical situations with assurance and competence.

- ## Importance of First Aid

First aid cannot be stressed in its value. First aid has the potential to save lives, prevent injuries from deteriorating, and encourage healing. Here are some of the key reasons why first aid is so important:

1. Saves lives: Providing first aid in an emergency might be the difference between life and death. Immediate

medical intervention may help to stabilize a person's condition until expert medical assistance arrives.

2. Prevents injuries from deteriorating: Prompt and good first aid may save an injury or disease from worsening. Stopping the bleeding, immobilizing a fractured bone, or providing an EpiPen, for example, may keep the situation from deteriorating.

3. Reduces pain and suffering: First aid may help the wounded or sick person feel better. Offering comfort and reassurance may also aid in the reduction of worry and tension.

4. Promotes healing: Proper first aid may assist in a speedier and more comfortable recovery from an accident or sickness.

5. Increases the odds of survival: In some medical situations, such as heart attacks or stroke, the chances of survival are much better if first aid is administered swiftly and efficiently.

6. Individuals are empowered: Learning first aid skills enables people to intervene in an emergency scenario and perhaps save lives. Knowing how to react to a medical emergency may help lessen worry and anxiety, as well as boost confidence and self-esteem.

Overall, first aid is an important skill that may make a big difference in an emergency. If you're looking for a unique way to express yourself creatively, here is the place to be.

• Legal and Ethical Considerations

When delivering first aid, there are legal and ethical factors that should be taken into mind. Here are some of the major legal and ethical factors to bear in mind:

1. Duty of Care: As a first aider, you have a legal responsibility to offer appropriate care to the wounded or unwell individual. Failure to offer reasonable care might result in legal responsibility.
2. permission: Before delivering first aid, you must get permission from the wounded or sick individual, or their legal representative if they are unable to grant consent themselves. It is necessary to clarify the nature of the first aid technique, and to respect the person's right to reject treatment.
3. Scope of Practice: It is crucial to recognize the boundaries of your first aid training and only offer treatment within your scope of practice. Attempting operations that are beyond your qualifications and skill might result in legal responsibility.
4. Confidentiality: Any information you receive about the wounded or unwell individual during the process of delivering first aid must be kept secret. Disclosure of

sensitive information might result in legal liability.

5. Good Samaritan Laws: Many countries have Good Samaritan laws that shield first aiders from legal responsibility if they perform in good faith and within the limits of their training. However, it is necessary to grasp the precise rules of the Good Samaritan Code in your area.

6. Cultural Considerations: When delivering first aid, it is crucial to be attentive to cultural variations and to respect the person's beliefs and values.

Overall, it is crucial to be aware of the legal and ethical implications while delivering first aid. Failure to comply to these concerns might result in legal responsibility or ethical issues.

2. Basic First Aid Procedures

Everyone should be familiar with the following first aid techniques:

1. Cardiopulmonary resuscitation (CPR): To sustain blood flow and oxygen to the brain and other essential organs, CPR involves chest compressions and rescue breathing. When someone is not breathing or has stopped heartbeat, CPR is performed.

2. Automated External Defibrillator (AED): In situations of abrupt cardiac arrest, an AED shocks the heart with electricity to restore a normal rhythm. Anyone, regardless of experience level, may use an AED.

3. Bleeding: Use a clean towel or bandage to provide direct pressure to the wound in cases of heavy bleeding. If at all feasible, elevate the injured limb while continuing to apply pressure until the bleeding stops.

4. Burns: To treat mild burns, run cold water over the area for a while. For more serious burns, you should get medical help right once and treat the area with a clean, non-fluffy covering.

5. A person who is choking and unable to breathe should be given the Heimlich technique, which involves stepping behind the individual, placing your arms around their waist, and quickly pushing up on their belly.

6. Fractures: Splint the injured limb if a person is believed to have a fracture in order to immobilize it and avoid additional harm. As soon as you can, get medical treatment.

7. Seizures: Preventing a person from being hurt during a seizure involves moving any adjacent items out of the way and supporting their head with a soft object. Never hold the individual down or put anything in their mouth.

These are only a few of the fundamental first aid methods that everyone should be familiar with. It's crucial to have the right first aid instruction and certification to understand these techniques and more complex ones.

- ## ABCs of First Aid (Airway, Breathing, Circulation)

The ABCs of first aid relate to the three key components that need to be examined and treated in an emergency situation: Airway, Breathing, and Circulation. Here's what each of these components means:

1. Airway: The airway is the passage that air flows through to reach the lungs. In an emergency case, it is necessary to check for any blockages in the airway, such as food, vomit, or a foreign item. If the

airway is clogged, it must be cleared before anything more may be done.

2. Breathing: Breathing is the process of breathing and exhaling air. whether the airway is clean, it is crucial to examine whether the individual is breathing. If the individual is not breathing, rescue breathing or CPR may be necessary to supply oxygen to the lungs and essential organs.

3. Circulation: Circulation refers to the flow of blood through the body. In an emergency scenario, it is necessary to look for evidence of circulation, such as a pulse or bleeding. If the individual is not breathing and has no pulse, CPR should be performed promptly to restore circulation.

Assessing the ABCs of first aid is a key step in any emergency scenario. It is crucial to respond promptly and efficiently to clear the airway, supply oxygen, and restore circulation as required. Remember, time is of the importance in a medical emergency, therefore it is crucial to respond swiftly and boldly to offer life-saving treatment.

- ## Bleeding and Shock

Bleeding and shock are two potentially life-threatening disorders that may arise as a consequence of injury or trauma. Here's everything you need to know about bleeding and shock:

1. Bleeding: Bleeding may be external or internal. External bleeding occurs when blood flows out of the body via an opening, such as a cut or wound. Internal bleeding occurs when blood collects within the body, such as from a fractured bone or organ injury. To reduce external bleeding, apply direct pressure to the area using a clean cloth or bandage. Elevate

the afflicted leg if feasible, and continue applying pressure until the bleeding stops. If the bleeding is significant or cannot be managed, get medical treatment immediately. indicators of internal bleeding include swelling, discomfort, and soreness in the afflicted location, as well as indicators of shock (see below).

2. Shock: Shock is a dangerous condition that may arise as a consequence of extreme bleeding or injury. Shock develops when there is not enough blood moving through the body to give oxygen to the important organs. Signs of shock include pale, chilly, clammy skin, fast breathing, a quick, weak pulse, confusion or disorientation, and loss of consciousness. To treat shock, lay the sufferer down with their legs raised above the level of their heart, if feasible. Cover them with a blanket to keep them warm, and seek medical assistance promptly.

It is crucial to act immediately to stop bleeding and manage shock in an emergency scenario. If you feel that someone is having serious bleeding or shock, contact for emergency medical help immediately.

- Burns and Scalds

Burns and scalds are injuries that come from exposure to heat or fire. Here's everything you need to know about treating burns and scalds:

1. First-degree burns: First-degree burns are mild burns that damage just the outer layer of skin. They are often characterized by redness, slight discomfort, and some edema. To treat a first-degree burn, run cold water over the injured area for several minutes. You may also use a cold compress to minimize swelling and soreness.   Over-the-counter   pain

medicines, such as acetaminophen or ibuprofen, may also help ease discomfort. Do not apply ice or butter on the burn, since this might make it worse.

2. Second-degree burns: Second-degree burns harm the outer and underlying layer of skin. They are characterized by redness, swelling, and the production of blisters. To cure a second-degree burn, run cold water over the injured area for several minutes. You may also use a cold compress to minimize swelling and soreness. Do not burst the blisters, since this might lead to infection. Over-the-counter pain medicines, such as acetaminophen or ibuprofen, may also help ease discomfort. Seek medical assistance if the burn is more than three inches in diameter, affects the face, hands, feet, or genitals, or is followed by fever or indications of infection.

3. Third-degree burns: Third-degree burns are the most serious form of burn and may harm all layers of the skin, as well as

the underlying tissue. They may seem burnt or blackened and may be accompanied by significant pain or numbness. Do not try to treat a third-degree burn yourself. Call for emergency medical help immediately.

4. Scalds: Scalds are burns that arise from exposure to hot liquids or steam. To treat a scald, remove any clothes or jewelry from the afflicted region and run cold water over the burn for several minutes. You may also use a cold compress to minimize swelling and soreness. If the scald is severe, get medical assistance immediately.

It is crucial to act immediately to treat burns and scalds to avoid infection and speed recovery. Seek medical treatment if the burn is serious or affects a big part of the body, or if you are unclear of how to treat the burn.

• Fractures and Dislocations

Fractures and dislocations are injuries that may happen from falls, accidents, or trauma. Here's what you need to know about treating fractures and dislocations:

1. Fractures: A fracture is a break in a bone. Symptoms may include discomfort, swelling, bruising, or deformity of the afflicted region. To cure a fracture, immobilize the damaged part by putting a splint or wrap over it. You may use a durable item, such as a rolled-up newspaper or a wooden stick, to form a splint. Elevate the afflicted region if feasible, and use ice to minimize swelling and discomfort. Seek medical assistance quickly, particularly if the fracture is serious or affects a joint, such as the hip or knee.

2. Dislocations: A dislocation occurs when a bone is displaced out of its usual position

at a joint. Symptoms may include discomfort, edema, or deformity of the afflicted joint. To treat a dislocation, immobilize the injured joint by putting a splint or wrap over it. You may use a durable item, such as a rolled-up newspaper or a wooden stick, to form a splint. Elevate the afflicted region if feasible, and use ice to minimize swelling and discomfort. Seek medical assistance quickly, particularly if the dislocation is severe or involves a joint, such as the shoulder or hip.

It is crucial to act swiftly to stabilize fractures and dislocations to avoid additional harm and facilitate healing. Seek medical assistance immediately if the fracture or dislocation is serious or affects a joint, or if you are unclear of how to manage the injury.

● Poisoning and Chemical Exposure

Poisoning and chemical exposure may happen through exposure to harmful compounds in the environment, such as home cleansers, insecticides, or carbon monoxide. Here's what you need to know about treating poisoning and chemical exposure:

1. Poisoning: If you believe someone has been poisoned, contact your local poison control center or emergency services immediately. Symptoms of poisoning may include nausea, vomiting, diarrhea, stomach discomfort, disorientation, or seizures. Do not induce vomiting unless told to do so by a medical practitioner. Keep the victim quiet and check their breathing and pulse until medical care comes.

2. Chemical exposure: If you come into touch with a poisonous chemical, remove any contaminated clothes and rinse the afflicted area with cold water for at least

20 minutes. If the chemical has spilled into the eyes, rinse them with cold water for at least 20 minutes. Seek medical treatment immediately if the exposure is significant, if the material is corrosive, or if you are suffering symptoms such as dizziness, trouble breathing, or chest discomfort.

Prevention is crucial when it comes to poisoning and chemical exposure. Keep harmful substances out of reach of children and pets, read product labels and utilize them according to instructions, and adequately ventilate places where chemicals are handled. If you feel a harmful or hazardous chemical has been swallowed or exposed, get medical care immediately.

- Choking and Suffocation

Choking and suffocation may arise from an item obstructing the airway or from a shortage of oxygen in the surroundings. Here's everything you need to know about treating choking and suffocation:

1. Choking: If someone is choking, urge them to cough and attempt to remove the item from their throat. If they are unable to cough, do the Heimlich technique by stepping behind them, positioning your fist just over their navel, and pushing upward and inside with a fast upward thrust. Repeat until the item is removed or the victim loses consciousness. If the victim loses consciousness, perform CPR immediately.

2. Suffocation: If someone is not breathing or has stopped breathing, notify emergency services immediately and begin CPR. Move the individual to a location with fresh air and, if feasible, open windows or doors to enhance

ventilation. If the individual is unconscious but still breathing, put them in the recovery position with their head inclined back and their chin up.

It is crucial to intervene swiftly in the event of choking or asphyxia. Learn the right skills for doing the Heimlich maneuver and CPR, and seek medical treatment promptly if the individual has lost consciousness or is not breathing. Take precautions to prevent choking and suffocating by avoiding tiny items that may be eaten and ensuring sufficient ventilation in regions with low oxygen levels.

- Heat and Cold Injuries

Heat and cold injuries may arise from prolonged exposure to high temperatures.

Here's what you need to know about treating heat and cold injuries:

1. Heat injuries: Heat injuries might include heat exhaustion, heat cramps, or heat stroke. Symptoms may include increased sweating, weakness, nausea, disorientation, or confusion. If someone is having signs of a heat injury, relocate them to a cooler environment and have them lay down. Apply cold, damp cloths to their skin, and have them drink cool water or a sports drink with electrolytes. Seek medical care promptly if the individual is having signs of heat stroke, such as a high body temperature, fast pulse, or unconsciousness.
2. Cold injuries: Cold injuries may include frostbite or hypothermia. Symptoms may include numbness, tingling, or discolouration of the skin. If someone is having signs of a cold injury, relocate them to a warmer environment and remove any damp clothes. Rewarm the injured region by immersing it in warm

water (104-108 degrees Fahrenheit) for 20-30 minutes or until the skin looks pink and flexible. Do not use hot water or direct heat sources, such as a heating pad or stove, to rewarm the afflicted region. Seek medical care promptly if the individual is exhibiting signs of hypothermia, such as shivering, disorientation, or loss of consciousness.

It is crucial to take care to prevent heat and cold injuries, such as keeping hydrated, wearing suitable clothes, and avoiding extended exposure to high temperatures. If you or someone else is suffering signs of a heat or cold injury, get medical assistance immediately to avoid severe consequences.

3. Medical Emergencies

Medical crises may encompass a broad variety of problems that need rapid medical intervention. Here are some frequent medical crises and what to do if you or someone else is experiencing them:

1. Heart attack: Symptoms of a heart attack may include chest discomfort, shortness of breath, nausea, or dizziness. If you or someone else is experiencing these symptoms, contact emergency services immediately and chew or swallow aspirin (if not allergic or instructed not to by a doctor). Do not wait getting medical help as quick treatment may save lives.
2. Stroke: Symptoms of a stroke may include abrupt numbness or weakness in the face, arm, or leg, disorientation, trouble speaking, or severe headache. If you or someone else is experiencing these symptoms, contact emergency services immediately. Note the timing of

commencement of symptoms, since time is crucial in deciding proper therapy.

3. Seizure: If someone is suffering a seizure, relocate them to a secure spot away from any things that might cause injury. Do not restrict the individual or put anything in their mouth. Call emergency services if the seizure lasts more than five minutes or if the individual is hurt during the seizure.

4. Allergic response: Symptoms of an allergic reaction may include hives, trouble breathing, or swelling of the face, lips, or tongue. If you or someone else is experiencing these symptoms, contact emergency services immediately and give an epinephrine auto-injector if available.

5. Overdose: If you believe someone has overdosed on drugs or medicine, contact emergency services immediately. Stay with the victim and check their breathing and pulse until medical aid comes.

It is crucial to keep cool and respond immediately in the event of a medical emergency. If you or someone else is suffering any indications of a medical emergency, contact emergency services immediately and get medical assistance as soon as possible.

- Heart Attack

A heart attack, also known as myocardial infarction, happens when the blood supply to the heart muscle is interrupted, generally by a blood clot. This may cause damage to the heart muscle and can be life-threatening. Here's what you need to know about spotting and reacting to a heart attack:

- Symptoms of a heart attack may include:

- Chest pain or discomfort, which may feel like pressure, squeezing, or fullness
- Pain or discomfort in the arms, neck, jaw, shoulder, or back
- Shortness of breath
- Sweating
- Nausea or vomiting
- Dizziness or lightheadedness
- Fatigue or weakness

If you or someone else is experiencing these symptoms, it is crucial to phone emergency services (such as 911 in the United States) immediately. Do not wait getting medical help, since timely treatment may save lives.

While waiting for emergency services to come, here are some things you may do to support the individual having the heart attack:

1. Have them sit down and relax in a comfortable posture.
2. If the individual is not allergic to aspirin and is not directed not to take it by a doctor, offer them one adult aspirin (325 mg) or four baby aspirins (81 mg each) to chew or swallow. This may assist to avoid blood clotting.
3. If the victim is unconscious and not breathing, administer CPR (cardiopulmonary resuscitation) until emergency personnel arrive.
4. Stay with the individual until emergency personnel come and offer any extra information they may need, such as drugs the person is taking or any prior medical issues.
5. Remember, identifying and reacting to the signs of a heart attack promptly may be essential in avoiding more damage to the heart and saving lives.

- Stroke

A stroke happens when there is an interruption in the blood flow to the brain, either due to a blood clot or bleeding in the brain. This may cause brain cells to die and can lead to major long-term impairment or even death. Recognizing the signs of a stroke and obtaining quick medical assistance is crucial in avoiding additional damage.

Here are some common signs of a stroke:

1. Sudden numbness or weakness in the face, arm, or leg, particularly on one side of the body Sudden disorientation, problems speaking or comprehending speech
2. Sudden difficulties seeing in one or both eyes
3. Sudden problem walking, dizziness, lack of balance or coordination
4. Sudden acute headache with no known reason

5. If you or someone else is experiencing these symptoms, contact emergency services (such as 911 in the United States) immediately. Every minute matters when it comes to treating a stroke.

6. While waiting for emergency services to come, here are some things you may do to support the individual having the stroke:

7. Have them sit down and relax in a comfortable posture.

8. If the victim is aware, attempt to keep them quiet and tell them that assistance is on the way.

9. Do not offer them anything to eat or drink, since this might interfere with medical therapy.

10. If the victim is unconscious and not breathing, administer CPR (cardiopulmonary resuscitation) until emergency personnel arrive.

Remember, identifying and reacting to the signs of a stroke promptly may be important in avoiding more damage to the brain and saving lives.

• Seizures and Epilepsy

Seizures are produced by aberrant electrical activity in the brain and may result in convulsions, loss of consciousness, and other symptoms. Epilepsy is a neurological condition that causes recurring seizures.

If you notice someone suffering a seizure, here are some measures you may do to help:

1. Stay with the individual and attempt to prevent them from harming themselves. Move any close things that might cause damage.
2. Place something soft, like a cushion or coat, beneath their head.

3. Loosen any tight clothes around their neck to make it simpler for them to breathe.

4. Do not attempt to hold the victim down or interrupt the seizure in any way.

5. Time the length of the seizure. If it lasts more than five minutes or if the individual has trouble breathing or displays indications of harm, contact emergency services (such as 911 in the United States) immediately.

6. After the seizure stops, turn the individual onto their side into the recovery position to avoid choking.

7. Stay with the individual until they completely recover or until emergency services come.

8. If someone has been diagnosed with epilepsy, it's crucial to know what to do in case of a seizure. In addition to the aforementioned stages, here are some extra points to bear in mind:

9. Make sure the individual takes their medicine as recommended.

10. Avoid causes that might produce seizures, such as stress, lack of sleep, or alcohol intake.

11. Encourage the individual to wear a medical alert bracelet or necklace that shows they have epilepsy.

12. Learn how to provide basic first aid for seizures and educate family and friends on what to do in case of an emergency.

13. Help the client construct an epilepsy management plan with their healthcare practitioner.

Remember, seizures may be terrifying and unexpected, but knowing what to do in an emergency can make a major difference in the result.

- ## Allergic Reactions and Anaphylaxis

An allergic response happens when the immune system overreacts to a chemical that is ordinarily innocuous, such as a specific meal, drug, or insect bite. Anaphylaxis is a serious and sometimes life-threatening allergic response that needs prompt medical intervention.

If you believe someone is suffering an allergic reaction, here are some things you may do to help:

1. Call emergency services immediately.
2. If the individual has an epinephrine auto-injector, such as an EpiPen, assist them use it as advised.
3. Have the sufferer lay down and raise their legs to promote blood flow.
4. Loosen any tight clothes around their neck to make it simpler for them to breathe.

5. Monitor the person's respiration, pulse, and state of awareness.
6. If the individual is vomiting or bleeding from the lips, flip them onto their side to avoid choking.
7. Stay with the individual until emergency personnel come and offer any extra information they may need, such as drugs the person is taking or any prior medical issues.
8. If the individual has a history of severe allergic responses, it's crucial that they have an epinephrine auto-injector with them at all times. In addition, individuals should wear a medical alert bracelet or necklace that shows they have a severe allergy.

Remember, allergic responses may be unexpected and even life-threatening. If you believe someone is suffering an allergic reaction, contact emergency services immediately and take actions to aid until medical help comes.

• Asthma and Breathing Difficulties

Asthma is a chronic respiratory disorder that may cause trouble breathing, wheezing, coughing, and chest tightness. Breathing problems may also be caused by other reasons such as allergies, infections, or other medical issues. Here are some things you may do to aid someone with asthma or breathing difficulties:

1. Encourage the individual to sit up straight and breathe gently and deeply.
2. If the individual has an inhaler, help them use it as instructed.
3. Loosen any tight clothes around their neck to make it simpler for them to breathe.
4. If the individual is suffering a severe asthma attack or having problems

breathing, contact emergency services (such as 911 in the United States) immediately.

5. If the victim is unconscious and not breathing, administer CPR (cardiopulmonary resuscitation) until emergency personnel arrive.

6. Stay with the individual until emergency personnel come and offer any extra information they may need, such as drugs the person is taking or any prior medical issues.

7. It's also vital to assist prevent asthma attacks and breathing problems by avoiding triggers such as allergies, tobacco, and pollution. Encourage the individual to engage with their doctor to build a treatment plan and to take their meds as recommended.

Remember, asthma and breathing issues may be severe and possibly life-threatening. If you believe someone is suffering an asthma attack or other breathing difficulties, take measures to aid and seek medical treatment if required.

• Diabetic Emergencies

Diabetes is a disorder in which the body is unable to appropriately manage blood sugar levels. This might lead to diabetic crises if blood sugar levels become too high or too low. Here are some actions you may take to aid someone facing a diabetic emergency:

1. whether the individual is cognizant and able to talk, inquire whether they have diabetes and if they have their diabetic supplies with them, such as insulin and a glucose meter.
2. If the individual is suffering hypoglycemia (low blood sugar), offer them a sweet drink or snack such as fruit juice, ordinary

soda, or candies. If the individual is unable to swallow, do not give them anything by mouth and seek medical treatment immediately.

3. If the client is having hyperglycemia (high blood sugar), advise them to drink water to keep hydrated.

4. If the individual is unconscious or unable to swallow, contact emergency services (such as 911 in the United States) immediately.

5. If the individual has an insulin pump and is suffering hypoglycemia, assist them unplug the pump.

6. Stay with the individual until emergency personnel come and offer any extra information they may need, such as drugs the person is taking or any prior medical issues.

7. It's also crucial to urge the individual to engage with their doctor to control their diabetes and to take their meds as advised. Encourage them to check their

blood sugar often and to have their diabetic supplies with them at all times.

Remember, diabetic crises may be severe and possibly life-threatening. If you believe someone is having a diabetic emergency, take measures to aid and seek medical treatment if required.

4. Specific First Aid Procedures

Here are some unique first aid practices you may encounter:

1. CPR (Cardiopulmonary resuscitation): CPR is a process used to restore breathing and circulation when a person's heart has stopped or they are not breathing. It includes chest compressions and rescue breaths.
2. Heimlich maneuver: The Heimlich technique is performed to aid a person who is choking on an item that is obstructing their airway. It entails putting pressure to the person's abdomen to assist release the item.
3. Bandaging: Proper bandaging may assist to halt bleeding and prevent a wound from infection. It's crucial to use a clean bandage and to apply pressure to the wound before bandaging.

4. Splinting: Splinting is used to stabilize a fractured bone or joint to avoid additional harm and minimize discomfort. It's crucial to apply a suitable splint and to prevent moving the damaged region.

5. Epinephrine auto-injector: An epinephrine auto-injector is used to treat severe allergic responses, often known as anaphylaxis. It releases a dosage of epinephrine, which may assist to expand the airways and relieve edema.

6. AED (Automated external defibrillator): An AED is a device used to restore a person's heart rhythm while they are suffering cardiac arrest. It sends a shock to the heart to assist it return to a regular rhythm.

7. Eye irrigation: Eye irrigation is used to drain foreign items or chemicals out of the eye. It entails using a clean, sterile fluid to cleanse the eye.

Remember, it's crucial to get medical treatment if someone is having a significant accident or medical emergency. These treatments may assist to stabilize a person until medical aid comes, but they are not a replacement for expert medical care.

• CPR (Cardiopulmonary Resuscitation)

CPR (Cardiopulmonary Resuscitation) is a lifesaving method used to resuscitate someone whose heart has stopped beating or who has stopped breathing. Here are the essential steps to administer CPR:

1. Check the situation for safety: Before commencing CPR, check sure the situation is safe and there are no risks that might put you or the victim in danger.
2. Check for responsiveness: Tap the person's shoulder and yell, "Are you okay?" to check whether they answer.

3. contact for help: If the individual does not reply, contact for emergency medical services (such as 911 in the United States) immediately.
4. Open the airway: Tilt the person's head back gently and elevate their chin to expose their airway.
5. Check for breathing: Look, listen, and feel for breathing. Look for chest movement, listen for breath sounds, and feel for breath on your cheek.
6. Start chest compressions: If the individual is not breathing or simply gasping, commence chest compressions. Place the heel of one hand on the middle of the person's chest and the second hand on top of the first. Push forcefully and rapidly, aiming for a pace of 100 to 120 compressions each minute.
7. provide rescue breaths: Pinch the person's nose closed and provide two rescue breaths. Watch for chest elevation with each inhalation.

8. Continue CPR: Alternate between chest compressions and rescue breaths, following the ratio of 30 compressions to 2 breaths.
9. Use an AED: If an automated external defibrillator (AED) is available, switch it on and follow the voice directions.
10. Continue CPR until aid arrives: Continue administering CPR until aid comes or the individual begins breathing on their own.

Remember, CPR may be a life-saving method, but it is crucial to be certified in CPR and refresh your skills frequently to ensure you can execute it effectively in an emergency circumstance.

- ## AED (Automated External Defibrillator) Use

An Automated External Defibrillator (AED) is a portable device that can evaluate the cardiac rhythm of a person who has collapsed and provide an electrical shock if required to restore a normal heartbeat. Here's everything you need to know about using an AED:

1. Call for emergency services: If you watch someone suddenly fall, immediately phone emergency services (such as 911 in the United States) to get aid on the way.
2. Locate and turn on the AED: If an AED is accessible, locate it and turn it on. Most AEDs will include voice instructions to take you through the processes.
3. Expose the chest and connect the pads: Remove any clothes covering the person's chest and adhere the pads to the person's bare chest. The AED will feature photos or

schematics demonstrating where to install the pads.

4. Analyze the heart rhythm: Press the analyze button on the AED, and wait for it to assess the person's heart beat. Make sure no one is touching the individual at this time.

5. Follow the AED's instructions: If the AED identifies a shockable rhythm, it will advise you to apply a shock. Make sure no one is touching the individual, and hit the shock button as indicated.

6. Begin CPR: After giving the shock, the AED will advise you to begin CPR. Follow the AED's voice instructions to give chest compressions and rescue breaths until emergency personnel arrive.

Remember, AEDs are meant to be used by anybody, regardless of training. The gadget will give audio instructions to help you through the processes, so do not be scared to use it if you come across someone who has collapsed.

- **First Aid for Children and Infants**

  delivering first aid to toddlers and newborns might need some different methods and procedures than delivering first aid to adults. Here are some things to bear in mind while delivering first aid to children and infants:

1. Adjust your strategy to the child's age and size: Children and newborns are smaller and more vulnerable than adults, thus it is vital to alter your approach appropriately. For example, while giving CPR, use two fingers instead of the heel of your hand for chest compressions for babies, and use just one hand for children between 1 and 8 years old.
2. Be conscious of the child's developmental stage: Children of various ages will have varying capacities and understandings of

what is occurring during a first aid emergency. For example, babies will not be able to explain their symptoms vocally, whereas older children may be able to provide you more specific information.

3. Consider the child's emotional state: Children may be terrified, unhappy, or in pain during a first aid crisis. Be careful to be cool and comforting, and explain what you are doing in a manner that they can comprehend. Use age-appropriate words and give comfort wherever feasible.

4. select suitable first aid items: Some first aid supplies may not be appropriate for children or newborns, so be sure to select products that are particularly developed for their size and requirements. For example, use a pediatric CPR mask while doing rescue breathing on a newborn or kid.

5. Be mindful of child-specific medical conditions: Children may experience medical disorders that are peculiar to their age, such as croup, febrile seizures,

or asthma. Be aware of these illnesses and their symptoms, and be prepared to administer proper first aid if required.

Remember, delivering first aid to children and babies may be tough, but it is crucial to stay calm and focused in order to offer the best treatment possible.

- ## First Aid for Pets

First aid for pets is a vital skill for pet owners and caretakers to have in case of emergency. Here are some basic suggestions for delivering first aid to pets:

1. Know your pet's usual behavior and behaviors. This might help you notice when anything is amiss and take action promptly.
2. Keep a pet first aid kit on hand. This should contain supplies like as gauze,

adhesive tape, scissors, antiseptic wipes, and a pet thermometer.

3. Know the location of the closest emergency veterinary clinic.

4. If your pet is hurt, keep cool and approach them carefully and softly. A scared or wounded pet may bite or scratch.

5. If your pet is bleeding, apply pressure to the area with a clean towel or gauze. If the bleeding does not cease after several minutes, seek veterinarian treatment.

6. If your pet is choking, attempt to remove the item if it is visible and can be safely recovered. If the item cannot be removed, seek veterinarian treatment immediately.

7. If your pet is suffering seizures, take them to a secure spot away from risks such as stairs or sharp objects. Do not attempt to restrain them or put anything in their mouth. Once the seizure has stopped, seek veterinarian treatment.

8. If your pet has consumed anything hazardous, call your veterinarian or a pet poison control hotline immediately.

Remember, offering first aid to pets is not a replacement for veterinarian treatment. Always seek veterinarian assistance for your pet as soon as possible in the case of an emergency or accident.

- ## First Aid for Sports Injuries

  Sports injuries are prevalent and may vary from minor bruising to major fractures. Here are some basic first aid methods that may be utilized for sports injuries:

1. Sprains and strains: Rest, ice, compression, and elevation (RICE) may help decrease swelling and discomfort. Rest the injured region, use ice to decrease swelling, apply a compression bandage to assist reduce swelling and support the injury, and elevate the damaged area to minimize swelling.

2. Fractures and dislocations: Do not try to move or correct the afflicted region. Immobilize the area with a splint or sling and seek medical assistance promptly.
3. Head injuries: If a head injury is suspected, immediately cease the activity and seek medical assistance. Keep the individual motionless and do not move them unless it is absolutely essential.
4. Heat exhaustion and heat stroke: Move the individual to a cooler spot, have them lay down and elevate their legs, and offer them cold water or sports drinks. If the individual develops indications of heat stroke, such as disorientation, convulsions, or loss of consciousness, seek medical assistance immediately.
5. Dehydration: Give the individual fluids, ideally water or sports drinks, and have them rest in a cool environment.
6. Cuts and abrasions: Clean the wound with soap and water, apply pressure to halt bleeding, and cover with a sterile bandage.

Remember, the best approach to avoid sports injuries is to properly warm up before physical activity, use appropriate protective gear, and employ right technique. If an accident does occur, it is crucial to seek medical assistance if required and to follow correct first aid protocols to minimize additional harm and facilitate recovery.

5. Preventing Injuries and Promoting Health

Preventing injuries and maintaining health is an essential element of first aid. Here are some recommendations for being safe and healthy:

1. Wear suitable protective gear: Depending on the activity, wearing protective gear including helmets, knee pads, and gloves may assist avoid injuries.
2. Warm up and stretch: Before participating in physical exercise, it is vital to warm up and stretch to avoid strains, sprains, and other injuries.
3. Stay hydrated: Drink lots of water before, during, and after strenuous exercise to avoid dehydration.
4. Know your limits: It is crucial to recognize your physical boundaries and not push yourself beyond them. Overexertion may lead to damage or sickness.

5. Practice good form and technique: Whether it's lifting weights or jogging, practicing proper form and technique will help avoid injuries.
6. Take pauses: If you are involved in a repetitive task, take regular rests to avoid overuse injuries.
7. Eat a balanced diet: Eating a balanced diet with lots of fruits, vegetables, and lean meats will help keep your body healthy and avoid disease.
8. Get adequate sleep: Getting enough sleep is vital for general health and may help avoid accidents and sickness.

By following these recommendations and exercising good habits, you may help avoid injuries and encourage a healthy lifestyle.

• Safety Precautions

Safety precautions are actions taken to avoid accidents, injuries, or other possible risks from happening. These measures may be taken in numerous circumstances, including at home, in the office, or during leisure activities. Here are some general safety measures that may be taken to lessen the chance of accidents or injuries:

1. Be alert of your surroundings: Keep an eye out for any risks in your surroundings, such as uneven ground, sharp objects, or unstable buildings.
2. Use protective equipment: Wear protective equipment such as helmets, gloves, or safety glasses while working with tools, machines, or chemicals.
3. Follow safety guidelines: Follow safety rules and instructions supplied by equipment makers, and be careful to operate equipment correctly and as intended.

4. Keep everything organized: Keep work environments tidy and clear of clutter to lessen the danger of tripping or falling.

5. Practice fire safety: Install smoke detectors in your house or business, and have a fire escape plan in place in case of an emergency.

6. Practice safe driving: Follow traffic regulations, wear seatbelts, and avoid distractions such as texting or using your phone while driving.

7. Practice proper food handling: Store food at safe temperatures, wash hands and surfaces regularly, and minimize cross-contamination when handling raw meats.

8. recognize your boundaries: Don't overexert yourself physically, and recognize your limits while engaging in sports or other physical activities.

These are only a few examples of safety procedures that may be followed to lessen the chance of accidents or injuries. Remember to constantly be vigilant of possible risks and take proper precautions to keep safe.

- ## Basic Hygiene and Sanitation

Basic hygiene and sanitation habits are crucial to preserving good health and limiting the spread of infectious illnesses. Here are some fundamental hygiene and sanitation habits that you may follow:

1. Wash your hands: Wash your hands often with soap and water for at least 20 seconds, particularly after using the restroom, before eating, and after coughing, sneezing, or blowing your nose.
2. Cover your mouth and nose: Cover your mouth and nose with a tissue or your elbow while coughing or sneezing to avoid the transmission of germs.

3. Keep surfaces clean: Clean and disinfect commonly touched surfaces such as doorknobs, light switches, and counters routinely.
4. Practice food safety: Wash fruits and vegetables well before eating, prepare meals to the right temperature, and minimize cross-contamination by using separate cutting boards and utensils for raw and cooked foods.
5. Maintain personal hygiene: Take a shower or bath frequently, wash your teeth twice a day, and keep your hair and nails clean.
6. Dispose of garbage properly: Dispose all garbage, including food waste and personal hygiene items, in approved containers and follow municipal waste disposal standards.
7. Drink clean water: Use clean water for drinking and cooking, and avoid consuming water from sources that may be polluted.

8. Practice safe sex: Use condoms during sexual activity to avoid the transmission of sexually transmitted illnesses.

These are just a few examples of fundamental hygiene and sanitation measures that may help you maintain good health and avoid the spread of infectious illnesses. Remember to constantly be attentive of your personal hygiene and take proper actions to keep a clean and healthy atmosphere.

• First Aid Kits and Supplies

A first aid kit is a collection of goods and equipment that is used to offer basic medical care for accidents or diseases that may occur at home, in the job, or when traveling. Here are some of the fundamental goods that should be included in a first aid kit:

1. Adhesive bandages in various sizes
2. Sterile gauze pads with sticky tape
3. Alcohol wipes or antiseptic solution
4. Non-latex gloves
5. Scissors and tweezers
6. Thermometer
7. Instant cold packs
8. Pain relievers such as acetaminophen or ibuprofen
9. Antihistamines for allergic responses
10. Prescription drugs (if required)

In addition to the aforementioned goods, you may also wish to take extra supplies that are particular to your requirements, such as an epinephrine auto-injector for severe allergic responses or a CPR face shield for doing CPR.

It's crucial to routinely inspect your first aid kit to verify that all materials are up to date and in excellent shape. Expired drugs and supplies should be disposed of appropriately and replaced as required. You may also want to consider attending a first aid course to learn basic first aid methods and how to utilize the equipment in your first aid kit successfully.

- Disaster Preparedness

Disaster preparation entails taking actions to prepare for and react to natural or man-made catastrophes such as earthquakes, hurricanes, floods, or terrorist attacks. Here are some things you may take to prepare for a disaster:

1. Make a plan: Create an emergency plan for you and your family that includes how

to contact each other, where to travel in case of evacuation, and what to do if you are separated.

2. Prepare a disaster kit: Prepare a catastrophe kit that contains supplies such as food, water, prescriptions, flashlights, and a first aid kit.

3. Stay informed: Stay informed about possible risks and calamities that may impact your region, and follow local news and weather alerts.

4. Secure your home: Secure your house by strengthening doors and windows, anchoring heavy furniture, and securing outside goods.

5. Evacuate if necessary: If you are advised to evacuate, follow evacuation instructions quickly and carry your disaster pack with you.

6. Learn basic first aid: Learn basic first aid skills so you can offer care to yourself or others in case of accident.

7. Practice emergency drills: Practice emergency drills with your family to

ensure everyone understands what to do in case of a tragedy.

8. Have emergency cash: Have a modest quantity of emergency cash handy in case ATMs or credit card systems are not operating.
9. Keep crucial papers safe: Keep crucial papers such as passports, birth certificates, and insurance policies in a waterproof container.
10. Remember that catastrophes may strike at any moment and being prepared can help you and your family remain safe during and after a disaster.

6. Conclusion

In conclusion, taking care to safeguard personal safety and well-being is vital in our daily lives. Basic hygiene and sanitation practices, first aid kits and supplies, and disaster preparedness are just a few examples of how we may be prepared and protect ourselves and our loved ones. By being attentive to our personal hygiene, keeping important medical supplies conveniently available, and preparing for likely disasters, we may minimize the likelihood of harm or sickness and be better equipped to meet unanticipated emergencies. Remember to continually stay informed, remain safe, and take care of yourself and others around you.In addition to the significance of getting expert medical treatment, it is also vital to maintain your first aid abilities up to date by routinely taking refresher classes or reading up on the newest knowledge. First aid practices may evolve over time, and remaining updated will help you deliver the most efficient assistance in an emergency.

It's also crucial to remember that first aid is not a replacement for emergency medical assistance. While first aid may give crucial help in the immediate aftermath of an accident or injury, it is not a replacement for skilled medical treatment. Seeking medical assistance as soon as possible after an accident or injury is vital to ensure that any underlying issues are adequately detected and treated.

Finally, it's important stressing that everyone may acquire first aid skills, regardless of age, background, or job. Basic first aid skills may make a major difference in an emergency scenario and can assist to save lives. By taking the time to learn first aid skills, you can become a valued asset in your community and help to make the world a safer place for everyone.

- **Recap of Important Points**

Sure, here's a review of the major things discussed:

1. Basic hygiene and sanitation behaviors, such as washing hands often, covering mouth and nose when coughing or sneezing, and keeping surfaces clean, are crucial to maintaining good health and reducing the spread of infectious illnesses.
2. A first aid kit should contain things such as adhesive bandages, sterile gauze pads, alcohol wipes, gloves, scissors, tweezers, thermometer, pain medicines, and prescription prescriptions if required.
3. Disaster preparation entails establishing a plan, assembling a disaster pack, staying informed, protecting your house, performing evacuation drills, learning basic first aid, and keeping essential papers secure.

Overall, completing these actions may help us be more prepared for unforeseen events, and secure our safety and well-being.

www.ingramcontent.com/pod-product-compliance
Lightning Source LLC
Chambersburg PA
CBHW071044220526
45467CB00004B/1673